My Health Care Diary

(Evergreen edition)

Developed by the team at

The Australian Allied Health Manual

in consultation with industry professionals.

This book has been developed based on personal and professional experience to improve communications between practitioners and patients, along with their carers and families.

AUSTRALIAN ALLIED HEALTH MANUAL

Better Business. Better Care.

www.alliedhealthmanual.com.au

PRINT ADDITIONAL TRACKING SHEETS AT HOME.

FREE DOWNLOAD AT www.alliedhealthmanual.com.au/diary

My Health Care Diary has been designed to assist not only you, but those most important around you in **your health journey**, including your Health Professionals, family and carers.

The Australian edition has been developed with common services in mind, meaning you can record your Medicare, DVA, NDIS details and more with ease.

This special evergreen edition has been developed with the ability for you start using it on any day of the year. Simply write your start date on the details page, find the page for your start date and loop back to use the remaining pages, or purchase the annual edition for a specific year.

The design and idea for this diary has not only come from years of knowledge in the health industry, and consultation with health professionals but also from the personal experience of dealing with up to 14 different health professionals all whilst trying to help our elderly parents navigate all their appointments. I personally was frustrated, as were my parents, going to an appointment and time and time again coming out saying ***"Oh I forgot to ask that" or "I don't remember what they said"***.

As you will see the book has comprehensive sections at the beginning allowing you to record everything about you and your medical history.

Each month begins with two tracking pages to record Blood Sugar Levels, Blood Pressure, Heart Rates and more.

We have also made available, via our website, free downloadable templates along with some extended versions of forms in the diary you may need extra of, to track more information and improve communications with your health care team.

We hope this diary helps you achieve **better care and better health through better communication**.

May '23

Su	M	Tu	W	Th	F	Sa
	1	2	3	4	5	6
7	8	9	10	11	12	13
14	15	16	17	18	19	20
21	22	23	24	25	26	27
28	29	30	31			

June '23

Su	M	Tu	W	Th	F	Sa
				1	2	3
4	5	6	7	8	9	10
11	12	13	14	15	16	17
18	19	20	21	22	23	24
25	26	27	28	29	30	

July '23

Su	M	Tu	W	Th	F	Sa
						1
2	3	4	5	6	7	8
9	10	11	12	13	14	15
16	17	18	19	20	21	22
23	24	25	26	27	28	29
30	31					

August '23

Su	M	Tu	W	Th	F	Sa
		1	2	3	4	5
6	7	8	9	10	11	12
13	14	15	16	17	18	19
20	21	22	23	24	25	26
27	28	29	30	31		

September '23

Su	M	Tu	W	Th	F	Sa
					1	2
3	4	5	6	7	8	9
10	11	12	13	14	15	16
17	18	19	20	21	22	23
24	25	26	27	28	29	30

October '23

Su	M	Tu	W	Th	F	Sa
1	2	3	4	5	6	7
8	9	10	11	12	13	14
15	16	17	18	19	20	21
22	23	24	25	26	27	28
29	30	31				

November '23

Su	M	Tu	W	Th	F	Sa
			1	2	3	4
5	6	7	8	9	10	11
12	13	14	15	16	17	18
19	20	21	22	23	24	25
26	27	28	29	30		

December '23

Su	M	Tu	W	Th	F	Sa
					1	2
3	4	5	6	7	8	9
10	11	12	13	14	15	16
17	18	19	20	21	22	23
24	25	26	27	28	29	30
31						

January '24

Su	M	Tu	W	Th	F	Sa
	1	2	3	4	5	6
7	8	9	10	11	12	13
14	15	16	17	18	19	20
21	22	23	24	25	26	27
28	29	30	31			

February '24

Su	M	Tu	W	Th	F	Sa
				1	2	3
4	5	6	7	8	9	10
11	12	13	14	15	16	17
18	19	20	21	22	23	24
25	26	27	28	29		

March '24

Su	M	Tu	W	Th	F	Sa
					1	2
3	4	5	6	7	8	9
10	11	12	13	14	15	16
17	18	19	20	21	22	23
24	25	26	27	28	29	30
31						

April '24

Su	M	Tu	W	Th	F	Sa
	1	2	3	4	5	6
7	8	9	10	11	12	13
14	15	16	17	18	19	20
21	22	23	24	25	26	27
28	29	30				

May '24

Su	M	Tu	W	Th	F	Sa
			1	2	3	4
5	6	7	8	9	10	11
12	13	14	15	16	17	18
19	20	21	22	23	24	25
26	27	28	29	30	31	

June '24

Su	M	Tu	W	Th	F	Sa
						1
2	3	4	5	6	7	8
9	10	11	12	13	14	15
16	17	18	19	20	21	22
23	24	25	26	27	28	29
30						

July '24

Su	M	Tu	W	Th	F	Sa
	1	2	3	4	5	6
7	8	9	10	11	12	13
14	15	16	17	18	19	20
21	22	23	24	25	26	27
28	29	30	31			

August '24

Su	M	Tu	W	Th	F	Sa
				1	2	3
4	5	6	7	8	9	10
11	12	13	14	15	16	17
18	19	20	21	22	23	24
25	26	27	28	29	30	31

September '24

Su	M	Tu	W	Th	F	Sa
1	2	3	4	5	6	7
8	9	10	11	12	13	14
15	16	17	18	19	20	21
22	23	24	25	26	27	28
29	30					

October '24

Su	M	Tu	W	Th	F	Sa
		1	2	3	4	5
6	7	8	9	10	11	12
13	14	15	16	17	18	19
20	21	22	23	24	25	26
27	28	29	30	31		

November '24

Su	M	Tu	W	Th	F	Sa
					1	2
3	4	5	6	7	8	9
10	11	12	13	14	15	16
17	18	19	20	21	22	23
24	25	26	27	28	29	30

December '24

Su	M	Tu	W	Th	F	Sa
1	2	3	4	5	6	7
8	9	10	11	12	13	14
15	16	17	18	19	20	21
22	23	24	25	26	27	28
29	30	31				

January '25

Su	M	Tu	W	Th	F	Sa
			1	2	3	4
5	6	7	8	9	10	11
12	13	14	15	16	17	18
19	20	21	22	23	24	25
26	27	28	29	30	31	

February '25

Su	M	Tu	W	Th	F	Sa
						1
2	3	4	5	6	7	8
9	10	11	12	13	14	15
16	17	18	19	20	21	22
23	24	25	26	27	28	

March '25

Su	M	Tu	W	Th	F	Sa
						1
2	3	4	5	6	7	8
9	10	11	12	13	14	15
16	17	18	19	20	21	22
23	24	25	26	27	28	29
30	31					

April '25

Su	M	Tu	W	Th	F	Sa
		1	2	3	4	5
6	7	8	9	10	11	12
13	14	15	16	17	18	19
20	21	22	23	24	25	26
27	28	29	30			

May '25

Su	M	Tu	W	Th	F	Sa
				1	2	3
4	5	6	7	8	9	10
11	12	13	14	15	16	17
18	19	20	21	22	23	24
25	26	27	28	29	30	31

June '25

Su	M	Tu	W	Th	F	Sa
1	2	3	4	5	6	7
8	9	10	11	12	13	14
15	16	17	18	19	20	21
22	23	24	25	26	27	28
29	30					

July '25

Su	M	Tu	W	Th	F	Sa
		1	2	3	4	5
6	7	8	9	10	11	12
13	14	15	16	17	18	19
20	21	22	23	24	25	26
27	28	29	30	31		

August '25

Su	M	Tu	W	Th	F	Sa
					1	2
3	4	5	6	7	8	9
10	11	12	13	14	15	16
17	18	19	20	21	22	23
24	25	26	27	28	29	30
31						

September '25

Su	M	Tu	W	Th	F	Sa
	1	2	3	4	5	6
7	8	9	10	11	12	13
14	15	16	17	18	19	20
21	22	23	24	25	26	27
28	29	30				

October '25

Su	M	Tu	W	Th	F	Sa
			1	2	3	4
5	6	7	8	9	10	11
12	13	14	15	16	17	18
19	20	21	22	23	24	25
26	27	28	29	30	31	

November '25

Su	M	Tu	W	Th	F	Sa
						1
2	3	4	5	6	7	8
9	10	11	12	13	14	15
16	17	18	19	20	21	22
23	24	25	26	27	28	29
30						

December '25

Su	M	Tu	W	Th	F	Sa
	1	2	3	4	5	6
7	8	9	10	11	12	13
14	15	16	17	18	19	20
21	22	23	24	25	26	27
28	29	30	31			

FULL NAME:

Date of Birth: / / Gender: Pronoun:

Address:

Phone:

Email:

Occupation:

I CARRY MEDICATION/EPI-PEN etc Yes/No:

Interpreter: Yes/No Language:

Preferred Hospital: Patient Number

Second Hospital: Patient Number

GP Name & Clinic:

GP Address:

GP Phone:

Preferred Pharmacy:

Pharmacy Phone:

Health Fund Name

Number: Ref:

Hospital Cover: Yes/No Extras Cover: Yes/No

Medicare Number: Ref: Exp:

DVA Number: Type: Gold/White/TPI (CIRCLE)

1st Emergency Contact:

1st Emergency Contact Phone:

2nd Emergency Contact:

2nd Emergency Contact Phone:

Additional Details & Important Contacts

List additional contacts & important details on this page

Work Cover Number:

Work Cover Case Manager:

Work Cover Case Manager Phone:

Preferred Transport Provider

Transport Provider Ref: Phone:

My Aged Care Ref: Phone:

NDIS Number:

TYPE: Self Managed/Plan Managed/NDIA Managed (CIRCLE)

NDIS Manager Name:

NDIS Manager Phone:

NDIS Manager Email:

Support Co-Ordinator Name:

Support Co-Ordinator Phone:

SMOKER: YES/NO: QTY ( ) Per DAY/WEEK

ALCOHOL: YES/NO: Std Drinks Per ( ) DAY/WEEK

SPECIALISTS INVOLVED IN MY CARE:

Eg Cardiologist/Oncologist/Neurologist/Physician/Orthopaedic Surgeon etc

NAME: PROFESSION:

LOCATION:

CONTACT NUMBER:

NAME: PROFESSION:

LOCATION:

CONTACT NUMBER:

NAME: PROFESSION:

LOCATION:

CONTACT NUMBER:

NAME: PROFESSION:

LOCATION:

CONTACT NUMBER:

NAME: PROFESSION:

LOCATION:

CONTACT NUMBER:

NAME: PROFESSION:

LOCATION:

CONTACT NUMBER:

NAME: PROFESSION:

LOCATION:

CONTACT NUMBER:

MY ALLIED HEALTH CARE TEAM:

Eg Physiotherapist/Podiatrist/Exercise Physiologist/Dietitian/Psychologist etc

NAME: PROFESSION:

LOCATION:

CONTACT NUMBER:

NAME: PROFESSION:

LOCATION:

CONTACT NUMBER:

NAME: PROFESSION:

LOCATION:

CONTACT NUMBER:

NAME: PROFESSION:

LOCATION:

CONTACT NUMBER:

NAME: PROFESSION:

LOCATION:

CONTACT NUMBER:

NAME: PROFESSION:

LOCATION:

CONTACT NUMBER:

NAME: PROFESSION:

LOCATION:

CONTACT NUMBER:

Do you have, or have you had, any of the following? Tick in box if yes.

AIDS/HIV Positive		Epilepsy		Osteoarthritis	
Alzheimer's Disease		Excessive Bleeding		Osteoporosis	
Anaemia		Excessive Thirst		Peripheral Vascular Disease	
Anaphylaxis		Fainting/Dizziness		Phlebitis	
Aneurysm		Frequent Cough		Polycystic Ovarian Syndrome	
Angina		Frequent Diarrhea		Pregnancy	
Ankylosing Spondylitis		Frequent Headaches		Prosthesis	
Arthritis/Gout		Gastric Sleeve/Band/ Bypass		Psoriatic Arthritis	
Artificial Heart Valve		Glaucoma		Psychiatric Care	
Artificial Joint		Gynaecological Issues		Radiation Treatment	
Asthma		Haemophilia		Recent Unexplained Weight Loss	
Blood Clots		Hay Fever		Reflux	
Blood Disease		Heart Attack/Failure		Reiter's Arthritis	
Blood Transfusion		Heart Disease		Renal Dialysis	
Breathing Problems		Heart Murmur		Respiratory Disorders	
Broken Bones		Heart Pacemaker		Rheumatic Fever	
Bruise Easily		Hepatitis A		Rheumatoid Arthritis	
Cancer		Hepatitis B		Scarlett Fever	
Cartilage Injury		Hepatitis C		Shingles	
Chemotherapy		Herpes		Sickle Cell Disease	
Chest Injury		High Blood Pressure		Sinus Trouble	
Chronic Pain		High Cholesterol		Skin Disorder	
Coeliac Disease		Hives or rash		Spina Bifida	
Cold Sores		Hypoglycaemia		Spinal Fracture/Trauma	
Congenital Heart Disorder		Infectious Disease		Stomach/Intestinal Disease	
Convulsions		Inflammatory Bowel Disease (IBD)		Stroke	
Cortisone Injection		Irregular Heartbeat		Swelling of limbs	
Crohn's Disease		Irritable Bowel Syndrome		Thyroid Disease	
Diabetes Type 1		Kidney Issues/Disease		Tonsilitis	
Diabetes Type 2		Leukemia		Tuberculosis	
Disc Problems		Ligament Injuries		Tumours/Growths	
Dislocations		Liver Issues/Disease		Ulcers	
Drug Addiction		Low Blood Pressure		Varicose Veins	
Easily Winded		Lung issues/Disease		Venereal Disease	
Emphysema		Mental Health Condition		Yellow Jaundice	

ALLERGY & INTOLLERANCE INFORMATION

ALLERGIC OR INTOLLERANT TO	NOTES (INCLUDING REACTION & TREATMENT)	TREATMENT (MEDICATION, EPI PEN ETC)

VACCINATION HISTORY

WHEN	WHAT	WHERE

SURGICAL HISTORY

DATE OF SURGERY	TYPE OF SURGERY	NOTES

SURGICAL HISTORY

DATE OF SURGERY	TYPE OF SURGERY	NOTES

FAMILY HISTORY

	Arthritis	Cancer	Diabetes	Genetic Disorder	Heart Condition	Lung Disease	Mental Illness	Stroke
Father								
	Details							
Mother								
	Details							
Siblings								
	Details							
Grandparents								
	Details							
Spouse								
	Details							
Other Family								
	Details							

MEDICATION

Medication	Dosage	DAY								WHEN				START DATE	FINISH DATE
		As Required	Sunday	Monday	Tuesday	Wednesday	Thursday	Friday	Saturday	Morning	Afternoon	Evening	Night		
Details/Reason for taking															
Details/Reason for taking															
Details/Reason for taking															
Details/Reason for taking															
Details/Reason for taking															
Details/Reason for taking															
Details/Reason for taking															
Details/Reason for taking															
Details/Reason for taking															
Details/Reason for taking															
Details/Reason for taking															
Details/Reason for taking															
Details/Reason for taking															

MEDICATION

Medication	Dosage	DAY								WHEN				START DATE	FINISH DATE
		As Required	Sunday	Monday	Tuesday	Wednesday	Thursday	Friday	Saturday	Morning	Afternoon	Evening	Night		
Details/Reason for taking															
Details/Reason for taking															
Details/Reason for taking															
Details/Reason for taking															
Details/Reason for taking															
Details/Reason for taking															
Details/Reason for taking															
Details/Reason for taking															
Details/Reason for taking															
Details/Reason for taking															
Details/Reason for taking															
Details/Reason for taking															
Details/Reason for taking															

OTHER MEDICAL HISTORY

FLUID TRACKING

Download additional copies to print at home on our website.

BASIC FLUID TRACKER			BATHROOM VISITS	ACCIDENTAL LEAKS		STRONG URGE TO GO		ACTIVITY
Day	TIME	INTAKE	HOW MANY	Y	N	Y	N	
EXAMPLE		2 cups	✓✓	×			×	Playing Soccer
1	5am-11am							
	11am-5pm							
	5pm-11pm							
	11pm-5am							
2	5am-11am							
	11am-5pm							
	5pm-11pm							
	11pm-5am							
3	5am-11am							
	11am-5pm							
	5pm-11pm							
	11pm-5am							
4	5am-11am							
	11am-5pm							
	5pm-11pm							
	11pm-5am							
5	5am-11am							
	11am-5pm							
	5pm-11pm							
	11pm-5am							
6	5am-11am							
	11am-5pm							
	5pm-11pm							
	11pm-5am							
7	5am-11am							
	11am-5pm							
	5pm-11pm							
	11pm-5am							

DENTAL/ORAL HISTORY

Date of last visit to Dentist			
Date of last dental Xray			
Reason for last visit to dentist			
How often do you brush			
How often do you floss			
Have you had any of the following?	Y	N	DETAILS
Bad Breath			
Biting Fingernails			
Bleeding Gums			
Blisters			
Burning/Tingling on tongue			
Chewing on one side of mouth			
Clicking or Popping Jaw			
Dentures/False			
Dry Mouth			
Fillings or Crowns			
Food collection between teeth			
Grinding of Teeth			
Jaw pain			
Lip or cheek biting			
Loose teeth			
Mouth breathing			
Orthodontic treatment			
Pain when brushing teeth			
Periodontal treatment			
Sensitivities - cold/hot/ sweet			
Smoking			
Tender or swollen gums			
Wisdom Teeth Removed			
Other			

7 DAY BOWEL TRACKER

Basic Bowel Tracker		Hard	Soft	Watery	Blood	Mucous	Offen-sive	Details
1	Morning							
	Afternoon							
	Evening							
	Night							
2	Morning							
	Afternoon							
	Evening							
	Night							
3	Morning							
	Afternoon							
	Evening							
	Night							
4	Morning							
	Afternoon							
	Evening							
	Night							
5	Morning							
	Afternoon							
	Evening							
	Night							
6	Morning							
	Afternoon							
	Evening							
	Night							
7	Morning							
	Afternoon							
	Evening							
	Night							

MONTHLY TRACKER Blood Pressure (BP) - Heart Rate (HR) - Blood Sugar (BSL)

JAN	MORNING			AFTERNOON			EVENING			NIGHT		
	BP	HR	BSL	BP	HR	BSL	BP	HR	BSL	BP	HR	BSL
1												
2												
3												
4												
5												
6												
7												
8												
9												
10												
11												
12												
13												
14												
15												
16												
17												
18												
19												
20												
21												
22												
23												
24												
25												
26												
27												
28												
29												
30												
31												

MONTHLY TRACKER Track the hours slept, steps, hours of exercise etc

JAN	SLEEP & REST		ACTIVITY		MOOD				
	SLEEP	REST	TYPE	QTY					
1									
2									
3									
4									
5									
6									
7									
8									
9									
10									
11									
12									
13									
14									
15									
16									
17									
18									
19									
20									
21									
22									
23									
24									
25									
26									
27									
28									
29									
30									
31									

Not tracking BP or BSL? You can use the columns to track, Temp, Oxygen, Temperature and other information useful to you.

WEEK	1	2	3	4
Weight				
Chest				
Waist				
Hips				

1 January 20___

QUESTIONS FOR MY CARE TEAM?

Have you got your week planned?

2 January 20___

QUESTIONS FOR MY CARE TEAM?

RESPONSES & THINGS TO REMEMBER.

NEED MORE SPACE? USE THE NOTES SECTION AT THE BACK OF THIS DIARY

3 January 20___

QUESTIONS FOR MY CARE TEAM?

Did you exercise today? Write it down!

4 January 20___

Do you e

RESPONSES & THINGS TO REMEMBER.

NEED MORE SPACE? USE THE NOTES SECTION AT THE BACK OF THIS DIARY

5 January 20___

QUESTIONS FOR MY CARE TEAM?

Are your tracking your weight or measurements?

6 January 20___

QUESTIONS FOR MY CARE TEAM?

RESPONSES & THINGS TO REMEMBER.

NEED MORE SPACE? USE THE NOTES SECTION AT THE BACK OF THIS DIARY

7 January 20___

QUESTIONS FOR MY CARE TEAM?

Have you got your week planned?

8 January 20___

QUESTIONS FOR MY CARE TEAM?

RESPONSES & THINGS TO REMEMBER.

NEED MORE SPACE? USE THE NOTES SECTION AT THE BACK OF THIS DIARY

9 January 20___

QUESTIONS FOR MY CARE TEAM?

Have you recorded your BP rate?

10 January 20___

QUESTIONS FOR MY CARE TEAM?

RESPONSES & THINGS TO REMEMBER.

NEED MORE SPACE? USE THE NOTES SECTION AT THE BACK OF THIS DIARY

11 January 20___

QUESTIONS FOR MY CARE TEAM?

Have you tracked your mood?

12 January 20___

QUESTIONS FOR MY CARE TEAM?

RESPONSES & THINGS TO REMEMBER.

NEED MORE SPACE? USE THE NOTES SECTION AT THE BACK OF THIS DIARY

13 January 20___

QUESTIONS FOR MY CARE TEAM?

Do you need to track your fluids?

14 January 20___

QUESTIONS FOR MY CARE TEAM?

RESPONSES & THINGS TO REMEMBER.

NEED MORE SPACE? USE THE NOTES SECTION AT THE BACK OF THIS DIARY

15 January 20___

QUESTIONS FOR MY CARE TEAM?

Did you exercise today? Write it down!

16 January 20___

QUESTIONS FOR MY CARE TEAM?

RESPONSES & THINGS TO REMEMBER.

NEED MORE SPACE? USE THE NOTES SECTION AT THE BACK OF THIS DIARY

17 January 20___

QUESTIONS FOR MY CARE TEAM?

Are your tracking your weight or measurements?

18 January 20___

QUESTIONS FOR MY CARE TEAM?

RESPONSES & THINGS TO REMEMBER.

NEED MORE SPACE? USE THE NOTES SECTION AT THE BACK OF THIS DIARY

19 January 20___

QUESTIONS FOR MY CARE TEAM?

Do you need to record your Blood Sugar Levels?

20 January 20___

QUESTIONS FOR MY CARE TEAM?

RESPONSES & THINGS TO REMEMBER.

NEED MORE SPACE? USE THE NOTES SECTION AT THE BACK OF THIS DIARY

21 January 20___

QUESTIONS FOR MY CARE TEAM?

Are you recording your heart rate? Write it down!

22 January 20___

QUESTIONS FOR MY CARE TEAM?

RESPONSES & THINGS TO REMEMBER.

NEED MORE SPACE? USE THE NOTES SECTION AT THE BACK OF THIS DIARY

23 January 20___

QUESTIONS FOR MY CARE TEAM?

Have you tracked your mood?

24 January 20___

QUESTIONS FOR MY CARE TEAM?

RESPONSES & THINGS TO REMEMBER.

NEED MORE SPACE? USE THE NOTES SECTION AT THE BACK OF THIS DIARY

25 January 20___

QUESTIONS FOR MY CARE TEAM?

Have you recorded your BP rate?

26 January 20___

QUESTIONS FOR MY CARE TEAM?

RESPONSES & THINGS TO REMEMBER.

NEED MORE SPACE? USE THE NOTES SECTION AT THE BACK OF THIS DIARY

27 January 20___

QUESTIONS FOR MY CARE TEAM?

Have you kept a track of your sleep?

28 January 20___

QUESTIONS FOR MY CARE TEAM?

RESPONSES & THINGS TO REMEMBER.

NEED MORE SPACE? USE THE NOTES SECTION AT THE BACK OF THIS DIARY

29 January 20___

QUESTIONS FOR MY CARE TEAM?

Did you exercise today? Write it down!

30 January 20___

QUESTIONS FOR MY CARE TEAM?

RESPONSES & THINGS TO REMEMBER.

NEED MORE SPACE? USE THE NOTES SECTION AT THE BACK OF THIS DIARY

31 January 20___

QUESTIONS FOR MY CARE TEAM?

Have you tracked your mood?

NOTES

NEED MORE SPACE? USE THE NOTES SECTION AT THE BACK OF THIS DIARY

MONTHLY TRACKER Blood Pressure (BP) - Heart Rate (HR) - Blood Sugar (BSL)

FEB	MORNING			AFTERNOON			EVENING			NIGHT		
	BP	HR	BSL	BP	HR	BSL	BP	HR	BSL	BP	HR	BSL
1												
2												
3												
4												
5												
6												
7												
8												
9												
10												
11												
12												
13												
14												
15												
16												
17												
18												
19												
20												
21												
22												
23												
24												
25												
26												
27												
28												
29												
30												
31												

MONTHLY TRACKER

Track the hours slept, Number steps, hours of exercise etc

FEB	SLEEP & REST		ACTIVITY		MOOD				
	SLEEP	REST	TYPE	QTY					
1									
2									
3									
4									
5									
6									
7									
8									
9									
10									
11									
12									
13									
14									
15									
16									
17									
18									
19									
20									
21									
22									
23									
24									
25									
26									
27									
28									
29									
30									
31									

Not tracking BP or BSL etc? You can use the columns to track, Temp, Oxygen, Flow Rates and other information useful to you.

WEEK	1	2	3	4
Weight				
Chest				
Waist				
Hips				

1 February 20___

QUESTIONS FOR MY CARE TEAM?

Are you tracking your mood?

HAVE YOU THOUGHT ABOUT GIFTING A DIARY TO A FRIEND?

2 February 20___

QUESTIONS FOR MY CARE TEAM?

RESPONSES & THINGS TO REMEMBER.

NEED MORE SPACE? USE THE NOTES SECTION AT THE BACK OF THIS DIARY

3 February 20___

QUESTIONS FOR MY CARE TEAM?

Did you exercise today? Write it down!

4 February 20___

QUESTIONS FOR MY CARE TEAM?

RESPONSES & THINGS TO REMEMBER.

NEED MORE SPACE? USE THE NOTES SECTION AT THE BACK OF THIS DIARY

5 February 20___

QUESTIONS FOR MY CARE TEAM?

Are your tracking your weight or measurements?

6 February 20___

QUESTIONS FOR MY CARE TEAM?

RESPONSES & THINGS TO REMEMBER.

NEED MORE SPACE? USE THE NOTES SECTION AT THE BACK OF THIS DIARY

7 February 20___

QUESTIONS FOR MY CARE TEAM?

Have you got your week planned?

8 February 20___

QUESTIONS FOR MY CARE TEAM?

RESPONSES & THINGS TO REMEMBER.

NEED MORE SPACE? USE THE NOTES SECTION AT THE BACK OF THIS DIARY

9 February 20___

QUESTIONS FOR MY CARE TEAM?

Have you recorded your Blood pressure?

10 February 20___

QUESTIONS FOR MY CARE TEAM?

RESPONSES & THINGS TO REMEMBER.

NEED MORE SPACE? USE THE NOTES SECTION AT THE BACK OF THIS DIARY

11 February 20___

QUESTIONS FOR MY CARE TEAM?

Have you told your family where to find this diary?

12 February 20___

QUESTIONS FOR MY CARE TEAM?

RESPONSES & THINGS TO REMEMBER.

NEED MORE SPACE? USE THE NOTES SECTION AT THE BACK OF THIS DIARY

13 February 20___

QUESTIONS FOR MY CARE TEAM?

Do you need to track your fluids?

14 February 20___

QUESTIONS FOR MY CARE TEAM?

RESPONSES & THINGS TO REMEMBER.

NEED MORE SPACE? USE THE NOTES SECTION AT THE BACK OF THIS DIARY

15 February 20___

QUESTIONS FOR MY CARE TEAM?

Did you exercise today? Write it down!

16 February 20___

QUESTIONS FOR MY CARE TEAM?

RESPONSES & THINGS TO REMEMBER.

NEED MORE SPACE? USE THE NOTES SECTION AT THE BACK OF THIS DIARY

17 February 20___

QUESTIONS FOR MY CARE TEAM?

Are your tracking your weight or measurements?

18 February 20___

QUESTIONS FOR MY CARE TEAM?

RESPONSES & THINGS TO REMEMBER.

NEED MORE SPACE? USE THE NOTES SECTION AT THE BACK OF THIS DIARY

19 February 20___

QUESTIONS FOR MY CARE TEAM?

Do you need to record your Blood Sugar Levels?

20 February 20___

QUESTIONS FOR MY CARE TEAM?

RESPONSES & THINGS TO REMEMBER.

NEED MORE SPACE? USE THE NOTES SECTION AT THE BACK OF THIS DIARY

21 February 20___

QUESTIONS FOR MY CARE TEAM?

What are you grateful for today?

22 February 20___

QUESTIONS FOR MY CARE TEAM?

RESPONSES & THINGS TO REMEMBER.

NEED MORE SPACE? USE THE NOTES SECTION AT THE BACK OF THIS DIARY

23 February 20___

QUESTIONS FOR MY CARE TEAM?

Have you tracked your mood?

24 February 20___

QUESTIONS FOR MY CARE TEAM?

Need more tracking sheets? Visit our website.

NEED MORE SPACE? USE THE NOTES SECTION AT THE BACK OF THIS DIARY

25 February 20___

QUESTIONS FOR MY CARE TEAM?

Have you recorded your BP rate?

26 February 20___

QUESTIONS FOR MY CARE TEAM?

RESPONSES & THINGS TO REMEMBER.

NEED MORE SPACE? USE THE NOTES SECTION AT THE BACK OF THIS DIARY

27 February 20___

QUESTIONS FOR MY CARE TEAM?

Have you kept a track of your sleep?

28/29 February 20___

QUESTIONS FOR MY CARE TEAM?

RESPONSES & THINGS TO REMEMBER.

NEED MORE SPACE? USE THE NOTES SECTION AT THE BACK OF THIS DIARY

MONTHLY TRACKER Blood Pressure (BP) - Heart Rate (HR) - Blood Sugar (BSL)

MAR	MORNING			AFTERNOON			EVENING			NIGHT		
	BP	HR	BSL	BP	HR	BSL	BP	HR	BSL	BP	HR	BSL
1												
2												
3												
4												
5												
6												
7												
8												
9												
10												
11												
12												
13												
14												
15												
16												
17												
18												
19												
20												
21												
22												
23												
24												
25												
26												
27												
28												
29												
30												
31												

MONTHLY TRACKER
Track the hours slept, steps, hours of exercise etc

MAR	SLEEP & REST		ACTIVITY		MOOD				
	SLEEP	REST	TYPE	QTY					
1									
2									
3									
4									
5									
6									
7									
8									
9									
10									
11									
12									
13									
14									
15									
16									
17									
18									
19									
20									
21									
22									
23									
24									
25									
26									
27									
28									
29									
30									
31									

Not tracking BP or BSL etc? You can use the columns to track, Temp, Oxygen, Flow Rates and other information useful to you.

WEEK	1	2	3	4
Weight				
Chest				
Waist				
Hips				

1 March 20___

QUESTIONS FOR MY CARE TEAM?

Have you got your week planned?

2 March 20___

QUESTIONS FOR MY CARE TEAM?

RESPONSES & THINGS TO REMEMBER.

NEED MORE SPACE? USE THE NOTES SECTION AT THE BACK OF THIS DIARY

3 March 20___

QUESTIONS FOR MY CARE TEAM?

Did you exercise today? Write it down!

4 March 20___

QUESTIONS FOR MY CARE TEAM?

RESPONSES & THINGS TO REMEMBER.

NEED MORE SPACE? USE THE NOTES SECTION AT THE BACK OF THIS DIARY

5 March 20___

QUESTIONS FOR MY CARE TEAM?

Are your tracking your weight or measurements?

6 March 20___

QUESTIONS FOR MY CARE TEAM?

RESPONSES & THINGS TO REMEMBER.

NEED MORE SPACE? USE THE NOTES SECTION AT THE BACK OF THIS DIARY

7 March 20___

QUESTIONS FOR MY CARE TEAM?

Have you got your week planned?

8 March 20___

QUESTIONS FOR MY CARE TEAM?

RESPONSES & THINGS TO REMEMBER.

NEED MORE SPACE? USE THE NOTES SECTION AT THE BACK OF THIS DIARY

9 March 20___

QUESTIONS FOR MY CARE TEAM?

Have you recorded your BP rate?

10 March 20___

QUESTIONS FOR MY CARE TEAM?

Need more tracking forms? Download from our website.

NEED MORE SPACE? USE THE NOTES SECTION AT THE BACK OF THIS DIARY

11 March 20___

QUESTIONS FOR MY CARE TEAM?

Have you tracked your mood?

12 March 20___

QUESTIONS FOR MY CARE TEAM?

RESPONSES & THINGS TO REMEMBER.

NEED MORE SPACE? USE THE NOTES SECTION AT THE BACK OF THIS DIARY

13 March 20___

QUESTIONS FOR MY CARE TEAM?

Do you need to track your fluids?

14 March 20___

QUESTIONS FOR MY CARE TEAM?

RESPONSES & THINGS TO REMEMBER.

NEED MORE SPACE? USE THE NOTES SECTION AT THE BACK OF THIS DIARY

15 March 20____

QUESTIONS FOR MY CARE TEAM?

Did you exercise today? Write it down!

16 March 20___

QUESTIONS FOR MY CARE TEAM?

RESPONSES & THINGS TO REMEMBER.

NEED MORE SPACE? USE THE NOTES SECTION AT THE BACK OF THIS DIARY

17 March 20___

QUESTIONS FOR MY CARE TEAM?

Are your tracking your weight or measurements?

18 March 20___

QUESTIONS FOR MY CARE TEAM?

RESPONSES & THINGS TO REMEMBER.

NEED MORE SPACE? USE THE NOTES SECTION AT THE BACK OF THIS DIARY

19 March 20___

QUESTIONS FOR MY CARE TEAM?

Do you need to record your Blood Sugar Levels?

20 March 20___

QUESTIONS FOR MY CARE TEAM?

RESPONSES & THINGS TO REMEMBER.

NEED MORE SPACE? USE THE NOTES SECTION AT THE BACK OF THIS DIARY

21 March 20___

QUESTIONS FOR MY CARE TEAM?

Do you need to measure your HR? Write it down!

22 March 20___

QUESTIONS FOR MY CARE TEAM?

RESPONSES & THINGS TO REMEMBER.

NEED MORE SPACE? USE THE NOTES SECTION AT THE BACK OF THIS DIARY

23 March 20___

QUESTIONS FOR MY CARE TEAM?

Have you tracked your mood?

24 March 20___

QUESTIONS FOR MY CARE TEAM?

RESPONSES & THINGS TO REMEMBER.

NEED MORE SPACE? USE THE NOTES SECTION AT THE BACK OF THIS DIARY

25 March 20___

QUESTIONS FOR MY CARE TEAM?

Have you recorded your BP rate?

26 March 20___

QUESTIONS FOR MY CARE TEAM?

RESPONSES & THINGS TO REMEMBER.

NEED MORE SPACE? USE THE NOTES SECTION AT THE BACK OF THIS DIARY

27 March 20___

QUESTIONS FOR MY CARE TEAM?

Have you kept a track of your sleep?

28 March 20___

QUESTIONS FOR MY CARE TEAM?

RESPONSES & THINGS TO REMEMBER.

NEED MORE SPACE? USE THE NOTES SECTION AT THE BACK OF THIS DIARY

29 March 20___

QUESTIONS FOR MY CARE TEAM?

Did you exercise today? Write it down!

30 March 20___

QUESTIONS FOR MY CARE TEAM?

RESPONSES & THINGS TO REMEMBER.

NEED MORE SPACE? USE THE NOTES SECTION AT THE BACK OF THIS DIARY

31 March 20___

QUESTIONS FOR MY CARE TEAM?

Have you tracked your mood?

NOTES

NEED MORE SPACE? USE THE NOTES SECTION AT THE BACK OF THIS DIARY

MONTHLY TRACKER Blood Pressure (BP) - Heart Rate (HR) - Blood Sugar (BSL)

APR	MORNING			AFTERNOON			EVENING			NIGHT		
	BP	HR	BSL	BP	HR	BSL	BP	HR	BSL	BP	HR	BSL
1												
2												
3												
4												
5												
6												
7												
8												
9												
10												
11												
12												
13												
14												
15												
16												
17												
18												
19												
20												
21												
22												
23												
24												
25												
26												
27												
28												
29												
30												
31												

MONTHLY TRACKER Track the hours slept, steps, hours of exercise etc

APR	SLEEP & REST		ACTIVITY		MOOD				
	SLEEP	REST	TYPE	QTY					
1									
2									
3									
4									
5									
6									
7									
8									
9									
10									
11									
12									
13									
14									
15									
16									
17									
18									
19									
20									
21									
22									
23									
24									
25									
26									
27									
28									
29									
30									
31									

Not tracking BP or BSL etc? You can use the columns to track, Temp, Oxygen, Flow Rates and other information useful to you.

WEEK	1	2	3	4
Weight				
Chest				
Waist				
Hips				

1 April 20___

QUESTIONS FOR MY CARE TEAM?

Have you got your week planned?

2 April 20___

QUESTIONS FOR MY CARE TEAM?

RESPONSES & THINGS TO REMEMBER.

NEED MORE SPACE? USE THE NOTES SECTION AT THE BACK OF THIS DIARY

3 April 20___

QUESTIONS FOR MY CARE TEAM?

Did you exercise today? Write it down!

4 April 20___

QUESTIONS FOR MY CARE TEAM?

RESPONSES & THINGS TO REMEMBER.

NEED MORE SPACE? USE THE NOTES SECTION AT THE BACK OF THIS DIARY

5 April 20___

QUESTIONS FOR MY CARE TEAM?

Are your tracking your weight or measurements?

6 April 20___

QUESTIONS FOR MY CARE TEAM?

RESPONSES & THINGS TO REMEMBER.

NEED MORE SPACE? USE THE NOTES SECTION AT THE BACK OF THIS DIARY

7 April 20___

QUESTIONS FOR MY CARE TEAM?

Have you got your week planned?

8 April 20___

QUESTIONS FOR MY CARE TEAM?

RESPONSES & THINGS TO REMEMBER.

NEED MORE SPACE? USE THE NOTES SECTION AT THE BACK OF THIS DIARY

9 April 20___

QUESTIONS FOR MY CARE TEAM?

Have you recorded your BP rate?

10 April 20___

QUESTIONS FOR MY CARE TEAM?

RESPONSES & THINGS TO REMEMBER.

NEED MORE SPACE? USE THE NOTES SECTION AT THE BACK OF THIS DIARY

11 April 20___

QUESTIONS FOR MY CARE TEAM?

Have you tracked your mood?

12 April 20___

QUESTIONS FOR MY CARE TEAM?

RESPONSES & THINGS TO REMEMBER.

NEED MORE SPACE? USE THE NOTES SECTION AT THE BACK OF THIS DIARY

13 April 20___

QUESTIONS FOR MY CARE TEAM?

Do you need to track your fluids?

14 April 20___

QUESTIONS FOR MY CARE TEAM?

RESPONSES & THINGS TO REMEMBER.

NEED MORE SPACE? USE THE NOTES SECTION AT THE BACK OF THIS DIARY

15 April 20___

QUESTIONS FOR MY CARE TEAM?

Did you exercise today? Write it down!

16 April 20___

QUESTIONS FOR MY CARE TEAM?

Do your caregivers know where to find this diary?

NEED MORE SPACE? USE THE NOTES SECTION AT THE BACK OF THIS DIARY

17 April 20___

QUESTIONS FOR MY CARE TEAM?

Are your tracking your weight or measurements?

18 April 20___

QUESTIONS FOR MY CARE TEAM?

RESPONSES & THINGS TO REMEMBER.

NEED MORE SPACE? USE THE NOTES SECTION AT THE BACK OF THIS DIARY

19 April 20___

QUESTIONS FOR MY CARE TEAM?

Do you need to record your Blood Sugar Levels?

20 April 20___

QUESTIONS FOR MY CARE TEAM?

RESPONSES & THINGS TO REMEMBER.

NEED MORE SPACE? USE THE NOTES SECTION AT THE BACK OF THIS DIARY

21 April 20___

QUESTIONS FOR MY CARE TEAM?

Do you need to measure your HR? Write it down!

22 April 20___

QUESTIONS FOR MY CARE TEAM?

RESPONSES & THINGS TO REMEMBER.

NEED MORE SPACE? USE THE NOTES SECTION AT THE BACK OF THIS DIARY

23 April 20___

QUESTIONS FOR MY CARE TEAM?

Have you tracked your mood?

24 April 20___

QUESTIONS FOR MY CARE TEAM?

RESPONSES & THINGS TO REMEMBER.

NEED MORE SPACE? USE THE NOTES SECTION AT THE BACK OF THIS DIARY

25 April 20___

QUESTIONS FOR MY CARE TEAM?

Have you recorded your BP rate?

26 April 20___

QUESTIONS FOR MY CARE TEAM?

RESPONSES & THINGS TO REMEMBER.

NEED MORE SPACE? USE THE NOTES SECTION AT THE BACK OF THIS DIARY

27 April 20___

QUESTIONS FOR MY CARE TEAM?

Have you kept a track of your sleep?

28 April 20___

QUESTIONS FOR MY CARE TEAM?

RESPONSES & THINGS TO REMEMBER.

NEED MORE SPACE? USE THE NOTES SECTION AT THE BACK OF THIS DIARY

29 April 20___

QUESTIONS FOR MY CARE TEAM?

Did you exercise today? Write it down!

30 April 20___

QUESTIONS FOR MY CARE TEAM?

RESPONSES & THINGS TO REMEMBER.

NEED MORE SPACE? USE THE NOTES SECTION AT THE BACK OF THIS DIARY

MONTHLY TRACKER Blood Pressure (BP) - Heart Rate (HR) - Blood Sugar (BSL)

MAY	MORNING			AFTERNOON			EVENING			NIGHT		
	BP	HR	BSL	BP	HR	BSL	BP	HR	BSL	BP	HR	BSL
1												
2												
3												
4												
5												
6												
7												
8												
9												
10												
11												
12												
13												
14												
15												
16												
17												
18												
19												
20												
21												
22												
23												
24												
25												
26												
27												
28												
29												
30												
31												

MONTHLY TRACKER

Track the hours slept, steps, hours of exercise etc

MAY	SLEEP & REST		ACTIVITY		MOOD				
	SLEEP	REST	TYPE	QTY	☹	😢	😐	🙂	🤩
1									
2									
3									
4									
5									
6									
7									
8									
9									
10									
11									
12									
13									
14									
15									
16									
17									
18									
19									
20									
21									
22									
23									
24									
25									
26									
27									
28									
29									
30									
31									

Not tracking BP or BSL etc? You can use the columns to track, Temp, Oxygen, Flow Rates and other information useful to you.

WEEK	1	2	3	4
Weight				
Chest				
Waist				
Hips				

1 May 20___

QUESTIONS FOR MY CARE TEAM?

Have you got your week planned?

2 May 20___

QUESTIONS FOR MY CARE TEAM?

RESPONSES & THINGS TO REMEMBER.

NEED MORE SPACE? USE THE NOTES SECTION AT THE BACK OF THIS DIARY

3 May 20___

QUESTIONS FOR MY CARE TEAM?

Did you exercise today? Write it down!

4 May 20___

QUESTIONS FOR MY CARE TEAM?

RESPONSES & THINGS TO REMEMBER.

NEED MORE SPACE? USE THE NOTES SECTION AT THE BACK OF THIS DIARY

5 May 20___

QUESTIONS FOR MY CARE TEAM?

Are your tracking your weight or measurements?

6 May 20___

QUESTIONS FOR MY CARE TEAM?

RESPONSES & THINGS TO REMEMBER.

NEED MORE SPACE? USE THE NOTES SECTION AT THE BACK OF THIS DIARY

7 May 20___

QUESTIONS FOR MY CARE TEAM?

Have you got your week planned?

8 May 20___

QUESTIONS FOR MY CARE TEAM?

RESPONSES & THINGS TO REMEMBER.

NEED MORE SPACE? USE THE NOTES SECTION AT THE BACK OF THIS DIARY

9 May 20___

QUESTIONS FOR MY CARE TEAM?

Have you recorded your BP rate?

10 May 20___

QUESTIONS FOR MY CARE TEAM?

RESPONSES & THINGS TO REMEMBER.

NEED MORE SPACE? USE THE NOTES SECTION AT THE BACK OF THIS DIARY

11 May 20___

QUESTIONS FOR MY CARE TEAM?

Have you tracked your mood?

12 May 20___

QUESTIONS FOR MY CARE TEAM?

RESPONSES & THINGS TO REMEMBER.

NEED MORE SPACE? USE THE NOTES SECTION AT THE BACK OF THIS DIARY

13 May 20___

QUESTIONS FOR MY CARE TEAM?

Do you need to track your fluids?

14 May 20___

QUESTIONS FOR MY CARE TEAM?

RESPONSES & THINGS TO REMEMBER.

NEED MORE SPACE? USE THE NOTES SECTION AT THE BACK OF THIS DIARY

15 May 20___

QUESTIONS FOR MY CARE TEAM?

Did you exercise today? Write it down!

16 May 20___

QUESTIONS FOR MY CARE TEAM?

RESPONSES & THINGS TO REMEMBER.

NEED MORE SPACE? USE THE NOTES SECTION AT THE BACK OF THIS DIARY

17 May 20___

QUESTIONS FOR MY CARE TEAM?

Are your tracking your weight or measurements?

18 May 20___

Need more trackers? Download them free from our website.

RESPONSES & THINGS TO REMEMBER.

NEED MORE SPACE? USE THE NOTES SECTION AT THE BACK OF THIS DIARY

19 May 20___

QUESTIONS FOR MY CARE TEAM?

What are you grateful for today?

20 May 20___

QUESTIONS FOR MY CARE TEAM?

RESPONSES & THINGS TO REMEMBER.

NEED MORE SPACE? USE THE NOTES SECTION AT THE BACK OF THIS DIARY

21 May 20___

QUESTIONS FOR MY CARE TEAM?

Do you need to measure your HR? Write it down!

22 May 20___

QUESTIONS FOR MY CARE TEAM?

RESPONSES & THINGS TO REMEMBER.

NEED MORE SPACE? USE THE NOTES SECTION AT THE BACK OF THIS DIARY

23 May 20___

QUESTIONS FOR MY CARE TEAM?

Have you tracked your mood?

24 May 20___

QUESTIONS FOR MY CARE TEAM?

RESPONSES & THINGS TO REMEMBER.

NEED MORE SPACE? USE THE NOTES SECTION AT THE BACK OF THIS DIARY

25 May 20___

QUESTIONS FOR MY CARE TEAM?

Have you recorded your BP rate?

26 May 20___

QUESTIONS FOR MY CARE TEAM?

RESPONSES & THINGS TO REMEMBER.

NEED MORE SPACE? USE THE NOTES SECTION AT THE BACK OF THIS DIARY

27 May 20___

QUESTIONS FOR MY CARE TEAM?

Have you kept a track of your sleep?

28 May 20___

QUESTIONS FOR MY CARE TEAM?

RESPONSES & THINGS TO REMEMBER.

NEED MORE SPACE? USE THE NOTES SECTION AT THE BACK OF THIS DIARY

29 May 20___

QUESTIONS FOR MY CARE TEAM?

Did you exercise today? Write it down!

30 May 20___

QUESTIONS FOR MY CARE TEAM?

RESPONSES & THINGS TO REMEMBER.

NEED MORE SPACE? USE THE NOTES SECTION AT THE BACK OF THIS DIARY

31 May 20___

QUESTIONS FOR MY CARE TEAM?

Have you tracked your mood?

NOTES

NEED MORE SPACE? USE THE NOTES SECTION AT THE BACK OF THIS DIARY

MONTHLY TRACKER Blood Pressure (BP) - Heart Rate (HR) - Blood Sugar (BSL)

JUN	MORNING			AFTERNOON			EVENING			NIGHT		
	BP	HR	BSL	BP	HR	BSL	BP	HR	BSL	BP	HR	BSL
1												
2												
3												
4												
5												
6												
7												
8												
9												
10												
11												
12												
13												
14												
15												
16												
17												
18												
19												
20												
21												
22												
23												
24												
25												
26												
27												
28												
29												
30												
31												

MONTHLY TRACKER Track the hours slept, steps, hours of exercise etc

JUN	SLEEP & REST		ACTIVITY		MOOD				
	SLEEP	REST	TYPE	QTY	☹	😥	😐	🙂	🤩
1									
2									
3									
4									
5									
6									
7									
8									
9									
10									
11									
12									
13									
14									
15									
16									
17									
18									
19									
20									
21									
22									
23									
24									
25									
26									
27									
28									
29									
30									
31									

Not tracking BP or BSL etc? You can use the columns to track, Temp, Oxygen, Flow Rates and other information useful to you.

WEEK	1	2	3	4
Weight				
Chest				
Waist				
Hips				

1 June 20___

QUESTIONS FOR MY CARE TEAM?

Have you got your week planned?

2 May 20___

QUESTIONS FOR MY CARE TEAM?

RESPONSES & THINGS TO REMEMBER.

NEED MORE SPACE? USE THE NOTES SECTION AT THE BACK OF THIS DIARY

3 June 20___

QUESTIONS FOR MY CARE TEAM?

Did you exercise today? Write it down!

4 June 20___

QUESTIONS FOR MY CARE TEAM?

RESPONSES & THINGS TO REMEMBER.

NEED MORE SPACE? USE THE NOTES SECTION AT THE BACK OF THIS DIARY

5 June 20___

QUESTIONS FOR MY CARE TEAM?

Are your tracking your weight or measurements?

6 June 20___

QUESTIONS FOR MY CARE TEAM?

RESPONSES & THINGS TO REMEMBER.

NEED MORE SPACE? USE THE NOTES SECTION AT THE BACK OF THIS DIARY

7 June 20___

QUESTIONS FOR MY CARE TEAM?

Have you got your week planned?

8 June 20___

QUESTIONS FOR MY CARE TEAM?

RESPONSES & THINGS TO REMEMBER.

NEED MORE SPACE? USE THE NOTES SECTION AT THE BACK OF THIS DIARY

9 June 20___

QUESTIONS FOR MY CARE TEAM?

Have you recorded your BP rate?

10 June 20___

QUESTIONS FOR MY CARE TEAM?

RESPONSES & THINGS TO REMEMBER.

NEED MORE SPACE? USE THE NOTES SECTION AT THE BACK OF THIS DIARY

11 June 20___

QUESTIONS FOR MY CARE TEAM?

Have you tracked your mood?

12 June 20___

QUESTIONS FOR MY CARE TEAM?

RESPONSES & THINGS TO REMEMBER.

NEED MORE SPACE? USE THE NOTES SECTION AT THE BACK OF THIS DIARY

13 June 20___

QUESTIONS FOR MY CARE TEAM?

Do you need to track your fluids?

14 June 20___

QUESTIONS FOR MY CARE TEAM?

RESPONSES & THINGS TO REMEMBER.

NEED MORE SPACE? USE THE NOTES SECTION AT THE BACK OF THIS DIARY

15 June 20___

QUESTIONS FOR MY CARE TEAM?

Did you exercise today? Write it down!

16 June 20___

QUESTIONS FOR MY CARE TEAM?

RESPONSES & THINGS TO REMEMBER.

NEED MORE SPACE? USE THE NOTES SECTION AT THE BACK OF THIS DIARY

17 June 20___

QUESTIONS FOR MY CARE TEAM?

Are your tracking your weight or measurements?

18 June 20___

QUESTIONS FOR MY CARE TEAM?

RESPONSES & THINGS TO REMEMBER.

NEED MORE SPACE? USE THE NOTES SECTION AT THE BACK OF THIS DIARY

19 June 20___

QUESTIONS FOR MY CARE TEAM?

Do you need to record your Blood Sugar Levels?

20 June 20___

QUESTIONS FOR MY CARE TEAM?

RESPONSES & THINGS TO REMEMBER.

NEED MORE SPACE? USE THE NOTES SECTION AT THE BACK OF THIS DIARY

21 June 20___

QUESTIONS FOR MY CARE TEAM?

Do you need to measure your HR? Write it down!

22 June 20___

QUESTIONS FOR MY CARE TEAM?

RESPONSES & THINGS TO REMEMBER.

NEED MORE SPACE? USE THE NOTES SECTION AT THE BACK OF THIS DIARY

23 June 20___

QUESTIONS FOR MY CARE TEAM?

Have you tracked your mood?

24 June 20___

QUESTIONS FOR MY CARE TEAM?

RESPONSES & THINGS TO REMEMBER.

NEED MORE SPACE? USE THE NOTES SECTION AT THE BACK OF THIS DIARY

25 June 20___

QUESTIONS FOR MY CARE TEAM?

Have you recorded your BP rate?

26 June 20___

QUESTIONS FOR MY CARE TEAM?

RESPONSES & THINGS TO REMEMBER.

NEED MORE SPACE? USE THE NOTES SECTION AT THE BACK OF THIS DIARY

27 June 20___

QUESTIONS FOR MY CARE TEAM?

Have you kept a track of your sleep?

28 June 20___

QUESTIONS FOR MY CARE TEAM?

RESPONSES & THINGS TO REMEMBER.

NEED MORE SPACE? USE THE NOTES SECTION AT THE BACK OF THIS DIARY

29 June 20___

QUESTIONS FOR MY CARE TEAM?

Did you exercise today? Write it down!

30 June 20___

QUESTIONS FOR MY CARE TEAM?

RESPONSES & THINGS TO REMEMBER.

NEED MORE SPACE? USE THE NOTES SECTION AT THE BACK OF THIS DIARY

MONTHLY TRACKER Blood Pressure (BP) - Heart Rate (HR) - Blood Sugar (BSL)

JUL	MORNING			AFTERNOON			EVENING			NIGHT		
	BP	HR	BSL	BP	HR	BSL	BP	HR	BSL	BP	HR	BSL
1												
2												
3												
4												
5												
6												
7												
8												
9												
10												
11												
12												
13												
14												
15												
16												
17												
18												
19												
20												
21												
22												
23												
24												
25												
26												
27												
28												
29												
30												
31												

MONTHLY TRACKER Track the hours slept, steps, hours of exercise etc

JUL	SLEEP & REST		ACTIVITY		MOOD				
	SLEEP	REST	TYPE	QTY	☹	😢	😐	🙂	🤩
1									
2									
3									
4									
5									
6									
7									
8									
9									
10									
11									
12									
13									
14									
15									
16									
17									
18									
19									
20									
21									
22									
23									
24									
25									
26									
27									
28									
29									
30									
31									

Not tracking BP or BSL etc? You can use the columns to track, Temp, Oxygen, Flow Rates and other information useful to you.

WEEK	1	2	3	4
Weight				
Chest				
Waist				
Hips				

1 July 20___

QUESTIONS FOR MY CARE TEAM?

Have you got your week planned?

2 July 20___

QUESTIONS FOR MY CARE TEAM?

RESPONSES & THINGS TO REMEMBER.

NEED MORE SPACE? USE THE NOTES SECTION AT THE BACK OF THIS DIARY

3 July 20___

QUESTIONS FOR MY CARE TEAM?

Did you exercise today? Write it down!

4 July 20___

QUESTIONS FOR MY CARE TEAM?

RESPONSES & THINGS TO REMEMBER.

NEED MORE SPACE? USE THE NOTES SECTION AT THE BACK OF THIS DIARY

5 July 20___

QUESTIONS FOR MY CARE TEAM?

Are your tracking your weight or measurements?

6 July 20___

QUESTIONS FOR MY CARE TEAM?

RESPONSES & THINGS TO REMEMBER.

NEED MORE SPACE? USE THE NOTES SECTION AT THE BACK OF THIS DIARY

7 July 20___

QUESTIONS FOR MY CARE TEAM?

Have you got your week planned?

8 July 20___

QUESTIONS FOR MY CARE TEAM?

RESPONSES & THINGS TO REMEMBER.

NEED MORE SPACE? USE THE NOTES SECTION AT THE BACK OF THIS DIARY

9 July 20___

QUESTIONS FOR MY CARE TEAM?

Have you recorded your BP rate?

10 July 20___

QUESTIONS FOR MY CARE TEAM?

RESPONSES & THINGS TO REMEMBER.

NEED MORE SPACE? USE THE NOTES SECTION AT THE BACK OF THIS DIARY

11 July 20___

QUESTIONS FOR MY CARE TEAM?

Have you tracked your mood?

12 July 20___

QUESTIONS FOR MY CARE TEAM?

RESPONSES & THINGS TO REMEMBER.

NEED MORE SPACE? USE THE NOTES SECTION AT THE BACK OF THIS DIARY

13 July 20___

QUESTIONS FOR MY CARE TEAM?

Do you need to track your fluids?

14 July 20___

QUESTIONS FOR MY CARE TEAM?

RESPONSES & THINGS TO REMEMBER.

NEED MORE SPACE? USE THE NOTES SECTION AT THE BACK OF THIS DIARY

15 July 20___

QUESTIONS FOR MY CARE TEAM?

Did you exercise today? Write it down!

16 July 20___

QUESTIONS FOR MY CARE TEAM?

RESPONSES & THINGS TO REMEMBER.

NEED MORE SPACE? USE THE NOTES SECTION AT THE BACK OF THIS DIARY

17 July 20___

QUESTIONS FOR MY CARE TEAM?

Are your tracking your weight or measurements?

18 July 20___

QUESTIONS FOR MY CARE TEAM?

RESPONSES & THINGS TO REMEMBER.

NEED MORE SPACE? USE THE NOTES SECTION AT THE BACK OF THIS DIARY

19 July 20___

QUESTIONS FOR MY CARE TEAM?

Do you need to record your Blood Sugar Levels?

20 July 20___

QUESTIONS FOR MY CARE TEAM?

RESPONSES & THINGS TO REMEMBER.

NEED MORE SPACE? USE THE NOTES SECTION AT THE BACK OF THIS DIARY

21 July 20___

QUESTIONS FOR MY CARE TEAM?

Do you need to measure your HR? Write it down!

22 July 20___

QUESTIONS FOR MY CARE TEAM?

RESPONSES & THINGS TO REMEMBER.

NEED MORE SPACE? USE THE NOTES SECTION AT THE BACK OF THIS DIARY

23 July 20___

QUESTIONS FOR MY CARE TEAM?

Have you tracked your mood?

24 July 20___

QUESTIONS FOR MY CARE TEAM?

RESPONSES & THINGS TO REMEMBER.

NEED MORE SPACE? USE THE NOTES SECTION AT THE BACK OF THIS DIARY

25 July 20___

QUESTIONS FOR MY CARE TEAM?

Have you recorded your BP rate?

26 July 20___

QUESTIONS FOR MY CARE TEAM?

RESPONSES & THINGS TO REMEMBER.

NEED MORE SPACE? USE THE NOTES SECTION AT THE BACK OF THIS DIARY

27 July 20___

QUESTIONS FOR MY CARE TEAM?

Have you kept a track of your sleep?

28 July 20___

QUESTIONS FOR MY CARE TEAM?

RESPONSES & THINGS TO REMEMBER.

NEED MORE SPACE? USE THE NOTES SECTION AT THE BACK OF THIS DIARY

29 July 20___

QUESTIONS FOR MY CARE TEAM?

Did you exercise today? Write it down!

30 July 20___

QUESTIONS FOR MY CARE TEAM?

RESPONSES & THINGS TO REMEMBER.

NEED MORE SPACE? USE THE NOTES SECTION AT THE BACK OF THIS DIARY

31 July 20___

QUESTIONS FOR MY CARE TEAM?

Have you tracked your mood?

NOTES

NEED MORE SPACE? USE THE NOTES SECTION AT THE BACK OF THIS DIARY

MONTHLY TRACKER Blood Pressure (BP) - Heart Rate (HR) - Blood Sugar (BSL)

AUG	MORNING			AFTERNOON			EVENING			NIGHT		
	BP	HR	BSL	BP	HR	BSL	BP	HR	BSL	BP	HR	BSL
1												
2												
3												
4												
5												
6												
7												
8												
9												
10												
11												
12												
13												
14												
15												
16												
17												
18												
19												
20												
21												
22												
23												
24												
25												
26												
27												
28												
29												
30												
31												

MONTHLY TRACKER Track the hours slept, steps, hours of exercise etc

AUG	SLEEP & REST		ACTIVITY		MOOD				
	SLEEP	REST	TYPE	QTY	☹	😢	😐	🙂	🤩
1									
2									
3									
4									
5									
6									
7									
8									
9									
10									
11									
12									
13									
14									
15									
16									
17									
18									
19									
20									
21									
22									
23									
24									
25									
26									
27									
28									
29									
30									
31									

Not tracking BP or BSL etc? You can use the columns to track, Temp, Oxygen, Flow Rates and other information useful to you.

WEEK	1	2	3	4
Weight				
Chest				
Waist				
Hips				

1 August 20___

QUESTIONS FOR MY CARE TEAM?

Have you got your week planned?

2 August 20___

QUESTIONS FOR MY CARE TEAM?

RESPONSES & THINGS TO REMEMBER.

NEED MORE SPACE? USE THE NOTES SECTION AT THE BACK OF THIS DIARY

3 August 20___

QUESTIONS FOR MY CARE TEAM?

Did you exercise today? Write it down!

4 August 20___

Communication is key to better health outcomes.

RESPONSES & THINGS TO REMEMBER.

NEED MORE SPACE? USE THE NOTES SECTION AT THE BACK OF THIS DIARY

5 August 20___

QUESTIONS FOR MY CARE TEAM?

Are your tracking your weight or measurements?

6 August 20___

QUESTIONS FOR MY CARE TEAM?

RESPONSES & THINGS TO REMEMBER.

NEED MORE SPACE? USE THE NOTES SECTION AT THE BACK OF THIS DIARY

7 August 20___

QUESTIONS FOR MY CARE TEAM?

Have you got your week planned?

8 August 20___

QUESTIONS FOR MY CARE TEAM?

RESPONSES & THINGS TO REMEMBER.

NEED MORE SPACE? USE THE NOTES SECTION AT THE BACK OF THIS DIARY

9 August 20___

QUESTIONS FOR MY CARE TEAM?

Have you recorded your BP rate?

10 August 20___

QUESTIONS FOR MY CARE TEAM?

RESPONSES & THINGS TO REMEMBER.

NEED MORE SPACE? USE THE NOTES SECTION AT THE BACK OF THIS DIARY

11 August 20___

QUESTIONS FOR MY CARE TEAM?

Have you tracked your mood?

12 August 20___

QUESTIONS FOR MY CARE TEAM?

RESPONSES & THINGS TO REMEMBER.

NEED MORE SPACE? USE THE NOTES SECTION AT THE BACK OF THIS DIARY

13 August 20___

QUESTIONS FOR MY CARE TEAM?

Do you need to track your fluids?

14 August 20___

QUESTIONS FOR MY CARE TEAM?

RESPONSES & THINGS TO REMEMBER.

NEED MORE SPACE? USE THE NOTES SECTION AT THE BACK OF THIS DIARY

15 August 20___

QUESTIONS FOR MY CARE TEAM?

Did you exercise today? Write it down!

16 August 20___

QUESTIONS FOR MY CARE TEAM?

RESPONSES & THINGS TO REMEMBER.

NEED MORE SPACE? USE THE NOTES SECTION AT THE BACK OF THIS DIARY

17 August 20___

QUESTIONS FOR MY CARE TEAM?

Are your tracking your weight or measurements?

18 August 20___

QUESTIONS FOR MY CARE TEAM?

RESPONSES & THINGS TO REMEMBER.

NEED MORE SPACE? USE THE NOTES SECTION AT THE BACK OF THIS DIARY

19 August 20___

QUESTIONS FOR MY CARE TEAM?

Do you need to record your Blood Sugar Levels?

20 August 20___

QUESTIONS FOR MY CARE TEAM?

RESPONSES & THINGS TO REMEMBER.

NEED MORE SPACE? USE THE NOTES SECTION AT THE BACK OF THIS DIARY

21 August 20___

QUESTIONS FOR MY CARE TEAM?

Do you need to measure your HR? Write it down!

22 August 20___

QUESTIONS FOR MY CARE TEAM?

RESPONSES & THINGS TO REMEMBER.

NEED MORE SPACE? USE THE NOTES SECTION AT THE BACK OF THIS DIARY

23 August 20___

QUESTIONS FOR MY CARE TEAM?

Have you tracked your mood?

24 August 20___

QUESTIONS FOR MY CARE TEAM?

RESPONSES & THINGS TO REMEMBER.

NEED MORE SPACE? USE THE NOTES SECTION AT THE BACK OF THIS DIARY

25 August 20___

QUESTIONS FOR MY CARE TEAM?

Have you recorded your BP rate?

26 August 20___

QUESTIONS FOR MY CARE TEAM?

RESPONSES & THINGS TO REMEMBER.

NEED MORE SPACE? USE THE NOTES SECTION AT THE BACK OF THIS DIARY

27 August 20___

QUESTIONS FOR MY CARE TEAM?

Have you kept a track of your sleep?

28 August 20___

QUESTIONS FOR MY CARE TEAM?

RESPONSES & THINGS TO REMEMBER.

NEED MORE SPACE? USE THE NOTES SECTION AT THE BACK OF THIS DIARY

29 August 20___

QUESTIONS FOR MY CARE TEAM?

Did you exercise today? Write it down!

30 August 20___

QUESTIONS FOR MY CARE TEAM?

RESPONSES & THINGS TO REMEMBER.

NEED MORE SPACE? USE THE NOTES SECTION AT THE BACK OF THIS DIARY

31 August 20___

QUESTIONS FOR MY CARE TEAM?

Have you tracked your mood?

NOTES

NEED MORE SPACE? USE THE NOTES SECTION AT THE BACK OF THIS DIARY

MONTHLY TRACKER Blood Pressure (BP) - Heart Rate (HR) - Blood Sugar (BSL)

SEP	MORNING			AFTERNOON			EVENING			NIGHT		
	BP	HR	BSL	BP	HR	BSL	BP	HR	BSL	BP	HR	BSL
1												
2												
3												
4												
5												
6												
7												
8												
9												
10												
11												
12												
13												
14												
15												
16												
17												
18												
19												
20												
21												
22												
23												
24												
25												
26												
27												
28												
29												
30												
31												

MONTHLY TRACKER Track the hours slept, steps, hours of exercise etc

SEP	SLEEP & REST		ACTIVITY		MOOD				
	SLEEP	REST	TYPE	QTY	😠	😢	😐	🙂	🤩
1									
2									
3									
4									
5									
6									
7									
8									
9									
10									
11									
12									
13									
14									
15									
16									
17									
18									
19									
20									
21									
22									
23									
24									
25									
26									
27									
28									
29									
30									
31									

Not tracking BP or BSL etc? You can use the columns to track, Temp, Oxygen, Flow Rates and other information useful to you.

WEEK	1	2	3	4
Weight				
Chest				
Waist				
Hips				

1 September 20___

QUESTIONS FOR MY CARE TEAM?

Have you got your week planned?

2 September 20____

QUESTIONS FOR MY CARE TEAM?

RESPONSES & THINGS TO REMEMBER.

NEED MORE SPACE? USE THE NOTES SECTION AT THE BACK OF THIS DIARY

3 September 20___

QUESTIONS FOR MY CARE TEAM?

What made you smile today?

4 September 20___

QUESTIONS FOR MY CARE TEAM?

RESPONSES & THINGS TO REMEMBER.

NEED MORE SPACE? USE THE NOTES SECTION AT THE BACK OF THIS DIARY

5 September 20___

QUESTIONS FOR MY CARE TEAM?

Are your tracking your weight or measurements?

6 September 20___

QUESTIONS FOR MY CARE TEAM?

RESPONSES & THINGS TO REMEMBER.

NEED MORE SPACE? USE THE NOTES SECTION AT THE BACK OF THIS DIARY

7 September 20___

QUESTIONS FOR MY CARE TEAM?

Have you got your week planned?

8 September 20___

QUESTIONS FOR MY CARE TEAM?

RESPONSES & THINGS TO REMEMBER.

NEED MORE SPACE? USE THE NOTES SECTION AT THE BACK OF THIS DIARY

9 September 20___

QUESTIONS FOR MY CARE TEAM?

Have you recorded your BP rate?

10 September 20___

Track next years appointments at the book of this book.

RESPONSES & THINGS TO REMEMBER.

NEED MORE SPACE? USE THE NOTES SECTION AT THE BACK OF THIS DIARY

11 September 20___

QUESTIONS FOR MY CARE TEAM?

Have you tracked your mood?

12 September 20___

QUESTIONS FOR MY CARE TEAM?

RESPONSES & THINGS TO REMEMBER.

NEED MORE SPACE? USE THE NOTES SECTION AT THE BACK OF THIS DIARY

13 September 20___

QUESTIONS FOR MY CARE TEAM?

Do you need to track your fluids?

14 September 20___

Need additional tracking forms? Visit our website to download and print at home.

RESPONSES & THINGS TO REMEMBER.

NEED MORE SPACE? USE THE NOTES SECTION AT THE BACK OF THIS DIARY

15 September 20___

QUESTIONS FOR MY CARE TEAM?

Did you exercise today? Write it down!

16 September 20___

QUESTIONS FOR MY CARE TEAM?

RESPONSES & THINGS TO REMEMBER.

NEED MORE SPACE? USE THE NOTES SECTION AT THE BACK OF THIS DIARY

17 September 20___

QUESTIONS FOR MY CARE TEAM?

Are your tracking your weight or measurements?

18 September 20___

QUESTIONS FOR MY CARE TEAM?

RESPONSES & THINGS TO REMEMBER.

NEED MORE SPACE? USE THE NOTES SECTION AT THE BACK OF THIS DIARY

19 September 20___

QUESTIONS FOR MY CARE TEAM?

Do you need to record your Blood Sugar Levels?

20 September 20___

QUESTIONS FOR MY CARE TEAM?

RESPONSES & THINGS TO REMEMBER.

NEED MORE SPACE? USE THE NOTES SECTION AT THE BACK OF THIS DIARY

21 September 20___

QUESTIONS FOR MY CARE TEAM?

Do you need to measure your HR? Write it down!

22 September 20___

QUESTIONS FOR MY CARE TEAM?

RESPONSES & THINGS TO REMEMBER.

NEED MORE SPACE? USE THE NOTES SECTION AT THE BACK OF THIS DIARY

23 September 20___

QUESTIONS FOR MY CARE TEAM?

Have you tracked your mood?

24 September 20___

QUESTIONS FOR MY CARE TEAM?

RESPONSES & THINGS TO REMEMBER.

NEED MORE SPACE? USE THE NOTES SECTION AT THE BACK OF THIS DIARY

25 September 20___

QUESTIONS FOR MY CARE TEAM?

Have you recorded your BP rate?

26 September 20___

Great health outcomes, need great communication.

RESPONSES & THINGS TO REMEMBER.

NEED MORE SPACE? USE THE NOTES SECTION AT THE BACK OF THIS DIARY

27 September 20___

QUESTIONS FOR MY CARE TEAM?

Have you kept a track of your sleep?

28 September 20___

QUESTIONS FOR MY CARE TEAM?

RESPONSES & THINGS TO REMEMBER.

NEED MORE SPACE? USE THE NOTES SECTION AT THE BACK OF THIS DIARY

29 September 20___

QUESTIONS FOR MY CARE TEAM?

Did you exercise today? Write it down!

30 September 20___

QUESTIONS FOR MY CARE TEAM?

RESPONSES & THINGS TO REMEMBER.

NEED MORE SPACE? USE THE NOTES SECTION AT THE BACK OF THIS DIARY

MONTHLY TRACKER Blood Pressure (BP) - Heart Rate (HR) - Blood Sugar (BSL)

OCT	MORNING			AFTERNOON			EVENING			NIGHT		
	BP	HR	BSL	BP	HR	BSL	BP	HR	BSL	BP	HR	BSL
1												
2												
3												
4												
5												
6												
7												
8												
9												
10												
11												
12												
13												
14												
15												
16												
17												
18												
19												
20												
21												
22												
23												
24												
25												
26												
27												
28												
29												
30												
31												

MONTHLY TRACKER

Track the hours slept, steps, hours of exercise etc

OCT	SLEEP & REST		ACTIVITY		MOOD				
	SLEEP	REST	TYPE	QTY					
1									
2									
3									
4									
5									
6									
7									
8									
9									
10									
11									
12									
13									
14									
15									
16									
17									
18									
19									
20									
21									
22									
23									
24									
25									
26									
27									
28									
29									
30									
31									

Not tracking BP or BSL etc? You can use the columns to track, Temp, Oxygen, Flow Rates and other information useful to you.

WEEK	1	2	3	4
Weight				
Chest				
Waist				
Hips				

1 October 20___

QUESTIONS FOR MY CARE TEAM?

Have you got your week planned?

2 October 20___

QUESTIONS FOR MY CARE TEAM?

RESPONSES & THINGS TO REMEMBER.

NEED MORE SPACE? USE THE NOTES SECTION AT THE BACK OF THIS DIARY

3 October 20___

QUESTIONS FOR MY CARE TEAM?

Did you exercise today? Write it down!

4 October 20___

QUESTIONS FOR MY CARE TEAM?

RESPONSES & THINGS TO REMEMBER.

NEED MORE SPACE? USE THE NOTES SECTION AT THE BACK OF THIS DIARY

5 October 20___

QUESTIONS FOR MY CARE TEAM?

Are your tracking your weight or measurements?

6 October 20___

QUESTIONS FOR MY CARE TEAM?

RESPONSES & THINGS TO REMEMBER.

NEED MORE SPACE? USE THE NOTES SECTION AT THE BACK OF THIS DIARY

7 October 20___

QUESTIONS FOR MY CARE TEAM?

Have you got your week planned?

8 October 20___

QUESTIONS FOR MY CARE TEAM?

RESPONSES & THINGS TO REMEMBER.

NEED MORE SPACE? USE THE NOTES SECTION AT THE BACK OF THIS DIARY

9 October 20___

QUESTIONS FOR MY CARE TEAM?

Have you recorded your BP rate?

10 October 20___

QUESTIONS FOR MY CARE TEAM?

RESPONSES & THINGS TO REMEMBER.

NEED MORE SPACE? USE THE NOTES SECTION AT THE BACK OF THIS DIARY

11 October 20___

QUESTIONS FOR MY CARE TEAM?

Have you tracked your mood?

12 October 20___

QUESTIONS FOR MY CARE TEAM?

RESPONSES & THINGS TO REMEMBER.

NEED MORE SPACE? USE THE NOTES SECTION AT THE BACK OF THIS DIARY

13 October 20___

QUESTIONS FOR MY CARE TEAM?

Do you need to track your fluids?

14 October 20___

QUESTIONS FOR MY CARE TEAM?

RESPONSES & THINGS TO REMEMBER.

NEED MORE SPACE? USE THE NOTES SECTION AT THE BACK OF THIS DIARY

15 October 20___

QUESTIONS FOR MY CARE TEAM?

Did you exercise today? Write it down!

16 October 20___

QUESTIONS FOR MY CARE TEAM?

RESPONSES & THINGS TO REMEMBER.

NEED MORE SPACE? USE THE NOTES SECTION AT THE BACK OF THIS DIARY

17 October 20___

QUESTIONS FOR MY CARE TEAM?

Are your tracking your weight or measurements?

18 October 20___

QUESTIONS FOR MY CARE TEAM?

RESPONSES & THINGS TO REMEMBER.

NEED MORE SPACE? USE THE NOTES SECTION AT THE BACK OF THIS DIARY

19 October 20___

QUESTIONS FOR MY CARE TEAM?

Do you need to record your Blood Sugar Levels?

20 October 20___

QUESTIONS FOR MY CARE TEAM?

RESPONSES & THINGS TO REMEMBER.

NEED MORE SPACE? USE THE NOTES SECTION AT THE BACK OF THIS DIARY

21 October 20___

QUESTIONS FOR MY CARE TEAM?

Do you need to measure your HR? Write it down!

22 October 20___

QUESTIONS FOR MY CARE TEAM?

RESPONSES & THINGS TO REMEMBER.

NEED MORE SPACE? USE THE NOTES SECTION AT THE BACK OF THIS DIARY

23 October 20___

QUESTIONS FOR MY CARE TEAM?

Have you tracked your mood?

24 October 20___

QUESTIONS FOR MY CARE TEAM?

RESPONSES & THINGS TO REMEMBER.

25 October 20___

QUESTIONS FOR MY CARE TEAM?

Have you recorded your BP rate?

26 October 20___

QUESTIONS FOR MY CARE TEAM?

RESPONSES & THINGS TO REMEMBER.

NEED MORE SPACE? USE THE NOTES SECTION AT THE BACK OF THIS DIARY

27 October 20___

QUESTIONS FOR MY CARE TEAM?

Have you kept a track of your sleep?

28 October 20___

QUESTIONS FOR MY CARE TEAM?

RESPONSES & THINGS TO REMEMBER.

NEED MORE SPACE? USE THE NOTES SECTION AT THE BACK OF THIS DIARY

29 October 20___

QUESTIONS FOR MY CARE TEAM?

Did you exercise today? Write it down!

30 October 20___

QUESTIONS FOR MY CARE TEAM?

RESPONSES & THINGS TO REMEMBER.

NEED MORE SPACE? USE THE NOTES SECTION AT THE BACK OF THIS DIARY

31 October 20___

QUESTIONS FOR MY CARE TEAM?

Have you tracked your mood?

NOTES

NEED MORE SPACE? USE THE NOTES SECTION AT THE BACK OF THIS DIARY

MONTHLY TRACKER Blood Pressure (BP) - Heart Rate (HR) - Blood Sugar (BSL)

NOV	MORNING			AFTERNOON			EVENING			NIGHT		
	BP	HR	BSL	BP	HR	BSL	BP	HR	BSL	BP	HR	BSL
1												
2												
3												
4												
5												
6												
7												
8												
9												
10												
11												
12												
13												
14												
15												
16												
17												
18												
19												
20												
21												
22												
23												
24												
25												
26												
27												
28												
29												
30												
31												

MONTHLY TRACKER Track the hours slept, steps, hours of exercise etc

NOV	SLEEP & REST		ACTIVITY		MOOD				
	SLEEP	REST	TYPE	QTY					
1									
2									
3									
4									
5									
6									
7									
8									
9									
10									
11									
12									
13									
14									
15									
16									
17									
18									
19									
20									
21									
22									
23									
24									
25									
26									
27									
28									
29									
30									
31									

Not tracking BP or BSL etc? You can use the columns to track, Temp, Oxygen, Flow Rates and other information useful to you.

WEEK	1	2	3	4
Weight				
Chest				
Waist				
Hips				

1 November 20___

QUESTIONS FOR MY CARE TEAM?

Have you got your week planned?

2 November 20___

QUESTIONS FOR MY CARE TEAM?

RESPONSES & THINGS TO REMEMBER.

NEED MORE SPACE? USE THE NOTES SECTION AT THE BACK OF THIS DIARY

3 November 20___

QUESTIONS FOR MY CARE TEAM?

Did you exercise today? Write it down!

4 November 20___

QUESTIONS FOR MY CARE TEAM?

RESPONSES & THINGS TO REMEMBER.

NEED MORE SPACE? USE THE NOTES SECTION AT THE BACK OF THIS DIARY

5 November 20___

QUESTIONS FOR MY CARE TEAM?

Are your tracking your weight or measurements?

6 November 20___

QUESTIONS FOR MY CARE TEAM?

RESPONSES & THINGS TO REMEMBER.

NEED MORE SPACE? USE THE NOTES SECTION AT THE BACK OF THIS DIARY

7 November 20___

QUESTIONS FOR MY CARE TEAM?

Have you got your week planned?

8 November 20___

QUESTIONS FOR MY CARE TEAM?

RESPONSES & THINGS TO REMEMBER.

NEED MORE SPACE? USE THE NOTES SECTION AT THE BACK OF THIS DIARY

9 November 20___

QUESTIONS FOR MY CARE TEAM?

Have you recorded your BP rate?

10 November 20___

QUESTIONS FOR MY CARE TEAM?

Communication is the key to Better Care.

NEED MORE SPACE? USE THE NOTES SECTION AT THE BACK OF THIS DIARY

11 November 20___

QUESTIONS FOR MY CARE TEAM?

Have you tracked your mood?

12 November 20___

QUESTIONS FOR MY CARE TEAM?

RESPONSES & THINGS TO REMEMBER.

NEED MORE SPACE? USE THE NOTES SECTION AT THE BACK OF THIS DIARY

13 November 20___

QUESTIONS FOR MY CARE TEAM?

Do you need to track your fluids?

14 November 20___

QUESTIONS FOR MY CARE TEAM?

RESPONSES & THINGS TO REMEMBER.

NEED MORE SPACE? USE THE NOTES SECTION AT THE BACK OF THIS DIARY

15 November 20___

QUESTIONS FOR MY CARE TEAM?

Did you exercise today? Write it down!

16 November 20___

QUESTIONS FOR MY CARE TEAM?

RESPONSES & THINGS TO REMEMBER.

NEED MORE SPACE? USE THE NOTES SECTION AT THE BACK OF THIS DIARY

17 November 20___

QUESTIONS FOR MY CARE TEAM?

Are your tracking your weight or measurements?

18 November 20___

QUESTIONS FOR MY CARE TEAM?

RESPONSES & THINGS TO REMEMBER.

NEED MORE SPACE? USE THE NOTES SECTION AT THE BACK OF THIS DIARY

19 November 20___

QUESTIONS FOR MY CARE TEAM?

Do you need to record your Blood Sugar Levels?

20 November 20___

QUESTIONS FOR MY CARE TEAM?

RESPONSES & THINGS TO REMEMBER.

NEED MORE SPACE? USE THE NOTES SECTION AT THE BACK OF THIS DIARY

21 November 20___

QUESTIONS FOR MY CARE TEAM?

Do you need to measure your HR? Write it down!

22 November 20___

QUESTIONS FOR MY CARE TEAM?

RESPONSES & THINGS TO REMEMBER.

NEED MORE SPACE? USE THE NOTES SECTION AT THE BACK OF THIS DIARY

23 November 20___

QUESTIONS FOR MY CARE TEAM?

Have you tracked your mood?

24 November 20___

QUESTIONS FOR MY CARE TEAM?

RESPONSES & THINGS TO REMEMBER.

25 November 20___

QUESTIONS FOR MY CARE TEAM?

Have you recorded your BP rate?

26 November 20___

QUESTIONS FOR MY CARE TEAM?

RESPONSES & THINGS TO REMEMBER.

NEED MORE SPACE? USE THE NOTES SECTION AT THE BACK OF THIS DIARY

27 November 20___

QUESTIONS FOR MY CARE TEAM?

Have you kept a track of your sleep?

28 November 20___

Are you tracking next years appointments?

RESPONSES & THINGS TO REMEMBER.

NEED MORE SPACE? USE THE NOTES SECTION AT THE BACK OF THIS DIARY

29 November 20___

QUESTIONS FOR MY CARE TEAM?

Did you exercise today? Write it down!

30 November 20___

QUESTIONS FOR MY CARE TEAM?

RESPONSES & THINGS TO REMEMBER.

NEED MORE SPACE? USE THE NOTES SECTION AT THE BACK OF THIS DIARY

MONTHLY TRACKER Blood Pressure (BP) - Heart Rate (HR) - Blood Sugar (BSL)

DEC	MORNING			AFTERNOON			EVENING			NIGHT		
	BP	HR	BSL	BP	HR	BSL	BP	HR	BSL	BP	HR	BSL
1												
2												
3												
4												
5												
6												
7												
8												
9												
10												
11												
12												
13												
14												
15												
16												
17												
18												
19												
20												
21												
22												
23												
24												
25												
26												
27												
28												
29												
30												
31												

MONTHLY TRACKER Track the hours slept, steps, hours of exercise etc

DEC	SLEEP & REST		ACTIVITY		MOOD				
	SLEEP	REST	TYPE	QTY					
1									
2									
3									
4									
5									
6									
7									
8									
9									
10									
11									
12									
13									
14									
15									
16									
17									
18									
19									
20									
21									
22									
23									
24									
25									
26									
27									
28									
29									
30									
31									

Not tracking BP or BSL etc? You can use the columns to track, Temp, Oxygen, Flow Rates and other information useful to you.

WEEK	1	2	3	4
Weight				
Chest				
Waist				
Hips				

1 December 20___

QUESTIONS FOR MY CARE TEAM?

Have you got your week planned?

2 December 20___

QUESTIONS FOR MY CARE TEAM?

RESPONSES & THINGS TO REMEMBER.

NEED MORE SPACE? USE THE NOTES SECTION AT THE BACK OF THIS DIARY

3 December 20___

QUESTIONS FOR MY CARE TEAM?

Did you exercise today? Write it down!

4 December 20___

QUESTIONS FOR MY CARE TEAM?

RESPONSES & THINGS TO REMEMBER.

NEED MORE SPACE? USE THE NOTES SECTION AT THE BACK OF THIS DIARY

5 December 20___

QUESTIONS FOR MY CARE TEAM?

Are your tracking your weight or measurements?

6 December 20___

QUESTIONS FOR MY CARE TEAM?

RESPONSES & THINGS TO REMEMBER.

NEED MORE SPACE? USE THE NOTES SECTION AT THE BACK OF THIS DIARY

7 December 20___

QUESTIONS FOR MY CARE TEAM?

Have you got your week planned?

8 December 20___

QUESTIONS FOR MY CARE TEAM?

RESPONSES & THINGS TO REMEMBER.

NEED MORE SPACE? USE THE NOTES SECTION AT THE BACK OF THIS DIARY

9 December 20___

QUESTIONS FOR MY CARE TEAM?

Have you recorded your BP rate?

10 December 20___

QUESTIONS FOR MY CARE TEAM?

RESPONSES & THINGS TO REMEMBER.

NEED MORE SPACE? USE THE NOTES SECTION AT THE BACK OF THIS DIARY

11 December 20___

QUESTIONS FOR MY CARE TEAM?

Have you tracked your mood?

12 December 20___

QUESTIONS FOR MY CARE TEAM?

RESPONSES & THINGS TO REMEMBER.

NEED MORE SPACE? USE THE NOTES SECTION AT THE BACK OF THIS DIARY

13 December 20___

QUESTIONS FOR MY CARE TEAM?

Do you need to track your fluids?

14 December 20___

QUESTIONS FOR MY CARE TEAM?

RESPONSES & THINGS TO REMEMBER.

NEED MORE SPACE? USE THE NOTES SECTION AT THE BACK OF THIS DIARY

15 December 20____

QUESTIONS FOR MY CARE TEAM?

Did you exercise today? Write it down!

16 December 20___

QUESTIONS FOR MY CARE TEAM?

RESPONSES & THINGS TO REMEMBER.

NEED MORE SPACE? USE THE NOTES SECTION AT THE BACK OF THIS DIARY

17 December 20___

QUESTIONS FOR MY CARE TEAM?

Are your tracking your weight or measurements?

18 December 20___

QUESTIONS FOR MY CARE TEAM?

RESPONSES & THINGS TO REMEMBER.

NEED MORE SPACE? USE THE NOTES SECTION AT THE BACK OF THIS DIARY

19 December 20___

QUESTIONS FOR MY CARE TEAM?

Do you need to record your Blood Sugar Levels?

20 December 20___

QUESTIONS FOR MY CARE TEAM?

RESPONSES & THINGS TO REMEMBER.

NEED MORE SPACE? USE THE NOTES SECTION AT THE BACK OF THIS DIARY

21 December 20___

QUESTIONS FOR MY CARE TEAM?

Do you need to measure your HR? Write it down!

22 December 20___

QUESTIONS FOR MY CARE TEAM?

RESPONSES & THINGS TO REMEMBER.

NEED MORE SPACE? USE THE NOTES SECTION AT THE BACK OF THIS DIARY

23 December 20___

QUESTIONS FOR MY CARE TEAM?

Have you tracked your mood?

24 December 20___

QUESTIONS FOR MY CARE TEAM?

RESPONSES & THINGS TO REMEMBER.

NEED MORE SPACE? USE THE NOTES SECTION AT THE BACK OF THIS DIARY

25 December 20___

QUESTIONS FOR MY CARE TEAM?

Have you recorded your BP rate?

26 December 20___

QUESTIONS FOR MY CARE TEAM?

RESPONSES & THINGS TO REMEMBER.

NEED MORE SPACE? USE THE NOTES SECTION AT THE BACK OF THIS DIARY

27 December 20___

QUESTIONS FOR MY CARE TEAM?

Have you kept a track of your sleep?

28 December 20___

QUESTIONS FOR MY CARE TEAM?

RESPONSES & THINGS TO REMEMBER.

NEED MORE SPACE? USE THE NOTES SECTION AT THE BACK OF THIS DIARY

29 December 20___

QUESTIONS FOR MY CARE TEAM?

Did you exercise today? Write it down!

30 December 20___

QUESTIONS FOR MY CARE TEAM?

RESPONSES & THINGS TO REMEMBER.

NEED MORE SPACE? USE THE NOTES SECTION AT THE BACK OF THIS DIARY

31 December 20___

QUESTIONS FOR MY CARE TEAM?

Have you tracked your mood?

NOTES

NEED MORE SPACE? USE THE NOTES SECTION AT THE BACK OF THIS DIARY

NOTES

NOTES

NEED MORE SPACE? USE THE NOTES SECTION AT THE BACK OF THIS DIARY

Appointments & Reviews for my next diary

Date	Who	Details (For & Why)

Made in the USA
Monee, IL
04 November 2026

67387244R00233